CHAIR YOGA FOR WOMEN OVER 60

Discover Strength, Flexibility,peace, and embrace Joy

Helen Talbott

Copyright Page

Chair Yoga for Women Over 60: Discover Strength, Flexibility, Peace, and Embrace Joy

Copyright © 2024 Helen Talbott

Disclaimer

The information contained in this book is for educational and informational purposes only. It is not intended to be a substitute for professional medical advice, diagnosis, or treatment. Always consult with your doctor before beginning any new exercise program, especially if you have any health conditions. The author and publisher disclaim any responsibility for any adverse effects arising from the use of the information contained in this book.

Disclaimer Page

The information presented in this book, **Chair Yoga for Women Over 60: Discover Strength, Flexibility, Peace, and Embrace Joy**, is intended for educational and informational purposes only. It is not intended to be a substitute for professional medical advice, diagnosis, or treatment.

Always consult with your healthcare provider before starting any new exercise program, especially if you have any underlying health conditions. The author and publisher disclaim any responsibility for any adverse effects arising from the use of the information contained within this book.

It is important to note that individual results may vary, and what works for one person may not work for another. Please listen to your body and modify the exercises as needed to fit your individual needs and abilities.

If you experience any pain or discomfort while practicing chair yoga, stop immediately and consult with your doctor.

By using this book, you acknowledge and agree to the terms of this disclaimer.

Table of contents

About The author

Helen Talbott is a passionate advocate for empowering women to discover strength, flexibility, and joy through the transformative practice of chair yoga. Her own journey began when she sought a gentle yet effective way to improve her fitness and wellbeing. Chair yoga became her sanctuary, offering a gateway to rediscover her physical capabilities and cultivate inner peace.

Driven by a desire to share this transformative experience with others, Helen embarked on a mission to create accessible and inclusive yoga practices tailored specifically for women over 60. Her book, **Chair Yoga for Women Over 60: Discover Strength, Flexibility, Peace, and Embrace Joy**, reflects this dedication. It's not just a collection of poses; it's a heartfelt guide that empowers women to embrace their bodies, celebrate their resilience, and unlock a newfound sense of joy through mindful movement.

Helen's approach is infused with warmth, understanding, and a touch of humor. She believes that age is just a number, and chair yoga is a powerful tool for unlocking one's full potential at any stage in life.

Beyond the book:

- Helen actively leads chair yoga workshops and classes, creating supportive communities where women can connect, learn, and laugh together.
- She is a regular contributor to health and wellness publications, sharing her expertise and passion for accessible fitness.
- Helen's infectious enthusiasm and dedication inspire women to embrace their journeys and discover the vibrant possibilities that lie ahead.

Join Helen on her mission to empower women over 60 to embrace strength, flexibility, and joy. Step into your chair, open your heart, and discover the transformative power of chair yoga with Helen Talbott as your guide.

Chapter 1

Introduction

Have you ever dreamed of experiencing the joy and benefits of yoga, but thought your body wasn't ready for the mat? Well, throw away those worries and grab a sturdy chair, because you're about to embark on a journey of **discovery, rejuvenation, and empowerment** in the wonderful world of chair yoga!

Forget intimidating downward dogs and pretzel-like contortions. Chair yoga is designed specifically for you, the vibrant woman over 60 who yearns for **strength, flexibility, and inner peace**. Imagine **cultivating serenity** while comfortably seated, gently stretching your muscles, and **building core power** without putting strain on your joints. With chair yoga, **age becomes just a number**, replaced by a sense of **renewed vitality and endless possibilities**.

This book is your **personal guide** to unlocking the magic of chair yoga. Whether you're a seasoned athlete or a complete beginner, we'll **begin with gentle movements** and gradually progress, tailoring poses to **every ability and body type**. You'll learn how to **infuse mindfulness into your practice, reduce stress and anxiety**, and discover a **supportive community** of women sharing their own chair yoga journeys.

Prepare to:

- **Unleash your inner strength** with poses that build stability and confidence.
- **Unveil your flexibility** with gentle stretches that improve range of motion.
- **Discover peace and harmony** through calming breathing techniques and guided meditations.

- **Embrace joy and well-being** as you integrate chair yoga into your daily routine.

No matter what your goals or limitations, chair yoga has something to offer. So, open this book, grab your chair, and get ready to **unveil a vibrant new chapter in your life!**

Are you ready to join me on this exciting journey? Turn the page and let's begin!

Why Chair Yoga is Perfect for You: Strength, Flexibility, and Joy Beyond the Mat

Imagine a form of yoga that offers **strength, flexibility, and peace of mind**, all while remaining comfortably seated in a chair. Sounds too good to be true, right? Well, welcome to the **wonderful world of chair yoga**, a practice specifically designed for women over 60 like you!

Here's why chair yoga might be the perfect fit for you:

Accessibility for All: Forget the intimidating poses and floor exercises of traditional yoga. Chair yoga uses your trusty chair as a supportive prop, making it **ideal for women of all fitness levels and physical abilities**. Whether you're just starting out, have joint pain, or haven't exercised in a while, chair yoga allows you to **participate safely and effectively**.

Unlocking Hidden Strength: Don't underestimate the power of a seated pose! Chair yoga incorporates gentle yet effective movements that target your core, legs, arms, and shoulders, helping you **build strength and stability** without putting undue stress on your joints. You'll be surprised at what you can achieve while comfortably seated!

Boosting Flexibility: As we age, our bodies naturally tighten up. Chair yoga counteracts this by incorporating gentle stretches that improve your **range of motion and flexibility**. You'll find yourself reaching further, bending deeper, and feeling more limber with each practice.

Finding Serenity Amidst Life's Busy-ness: Chair yoga doesn't just benefit your body; it's a haven for your mind and spirit. By incorporating mindful breathing techniques and guided meditations, you'll learn to **reduce stress, manage anxiety, and cultivate inner peace**, even in the midst of your busy life.

Embracing Joyful Movement: Forget the image of rigid poses and forced contortions. Chair yoga is designed to be **enjoyable and**

uplifting. You'll experience the **joy of movement** as you flow through gentle sequences, feel the invigorating energy of gentle strength training, and discover the serenity of mindful breathing.

Building a Supportive Community: Chair yoga isn't just an individual practice; it's a chance to connect with other women who understand your unique needs and goals. Whether you join a local class or practice online, you'll find a community of supportive women who will encourage and motivate you on your journey.

Remember, chair yoga is about more than just physical postures. It's about **empowering yourself**, discovering your inner strength, and **embracing a life filled with joy and well-being**. So, grab your chair, take a deep breath, and get ready to embark on a transformative journey that starts right now!

The Incredible Benefits You'll Reap: Beyond Strength and Flexibility with Chair Yoga

Chair yoga isn't just a gentle exercise routine; it's a **treasure trove of benefits** waiting to be unlocked! While building strength and flexibility are fantastic rewards, the magic of chair yoga goes far beyond the physical. Here's a glimpse of the incredible benefits you'll reap:

Enhanced Balance and Stability: Wobbly on your feet? Fear not! Chair yoga incorporates poses that challenge your balance in a safe and controlled environment, increasing your confidence and reducing your risk of falls. Imagine stepping out with newfound steadiness and enjoying activities you may have once hesitated to do.

Improved Pain Management: Whether you live with chronic pain or experience occasional aches, chair yoga can be your gentle ally. Specific poses and stretches can help manage and even reduce pain in your joints, muscles, and back, leaving you feeling more comfortable and mobile throughout the day.

Reduced Stress and Anxiety: Feeling overwhelmed by life's demands? Chair yoga offers a soothing escape. Deep breathing exercises and mindful movements help quiet your mind, melt away tension, and cultivate a sense of inner calm. You'll learn to manage stress more effectively and approach your day with greater peace of mind.

Boosted Energy and Mood: Feeling sluggish or down? Chair yoga can be your natural energy booster! The combination of gentle movement, focused breathing, and mindful presence revitalizes your body and lifts your spirits. You'll notice increased energy levels, improved sleep, and a more positive outlook on life.

Sharpened Cognitive Function: Don't underestimate the power of chair yoga for your brain! Studies show that yoga can improve memory, focus, and cognitive function. As you flow through sequences and focus on your breath, you'll be stimulating your mind and keeping it sharp for years to come.

Greater Confidence and Self-Esteem: As you experience the positive changes in your body and mind, your confidence will naturally blossom. The sense of accomplishment from mastering new poses, the increased strength and flexibility, and the overall improved well-being will contribute to a more positive self-image and a newfound sense of empowerment.

Enhanced Social Connection: Feeling isolated or disconnected? Chair yoga offers a wonderful opportunity to connect with other women like you. Whether you choose online classes or local groups, you'll find a supportive community of individuals sharing their experiences and encouraging each other on their journeys.

These are just a few of the incredible benefits waiting to be discovered with chair yoga. Remember, it's not about pushing your limits or achieving perfection; it's about celebrating your body, cultivating your well-being, and embracing a life filled with joy, strength, and newfound possibilities. So, take the first step towards a healthier and happier you – one gentle pose at a time!

Yoga myths debunked for the discerning woman over 60

Myth 1: You Need to Be Flexible to Do Yoga

This is probably the most common misconception about yoga! Yoga isn't a competition about who can twist themselves into the pretzel-iest shape. Chair yoga, in particular, is designed for **accessibility and inclusivity**, meaning it's perfect for beginners and those with limited flexibility. The focus is on gentle movements, breathwork, and mindfulness, making it **enjoyable and beneficial for everyone**, regardless of their current physical abilities.

Myth 2: Yoga is Just for Young People

Absolutely not! Chair yoga is specifically designed for individuals like you, **women over 60 who crave a gentle yet effective way to improve their well-being**. In fact, the practice offers numerous benefits that are particularly valuable for mature adults, such as **improved balance, increased strength, and reduced stress**. You'll find a welcoming community of women from all walks of life in chair yoga classes, proving that yoga is ageless and enriching for everyone.

Myth 3: Chair Yoga Isn't a Real Workout

While chair yoga might not get your heart rate soaring like a Zumba class, it doesn't mean it's not a workout! Don't underestimate the power of gentle, targeted movements. Chair yoga effectively **engages your core, strengthens your muscles, and improves your range of motion**, all while being kind to your joints. You'll be surprised at how energized and accomplished you feel after a chair yoga session, proving that a powerful workout doesn't have to be jarring or extreme.

Myth 4: You Need Expensive Equipment to Do Yoga

All you need for chair yoga is a sturdy chair and yourself! No fancy mats, blocks, or straps are required. This makes it an **accessible and affordable way** to experience the benefits of yoga, regardless of your budget. You can even practice chair yoga from the comfort of your own home, using a dining chair or an armchair.

Myth 5: Yoga is a Religion

Yoga is an ancient practice with roots in Hindu philosophy, but it's not inherently religious. You can **fully participate in and reap the benefits of yoga without subscribing to any specific belief system.** Chair yoga focuses on the physical and mental aspects of the practice, offering stress reduction, improved flexibility, and a sense of well-being for individuals of all faiths and backgrounds.

So, there you have it! Don't let these common myths hold you back from experiencing the wonders of chair yoga. It's a practice designed for you, offering a wealth of benefits and a supportive community to help you on your journey to a healthier and happier you.

Embark on Your Chair Yoga Journey: The Essentials You Need

Ready to dive into the world of chair yoga and unlock its incredible benefits? Let's gather everything you need to get started comfortably and confidently:

Your Reliable Throne: The star of the show! Choose a **sturdy, armless chair** with a flat seat and a back that allows you to sit comfortably with your feet flat on the floor. Avoid swivel chairs or those with wheels for safety reasons.

Your Comfy Outfit: Dress in **loose-fitting, breathable clothing** that allows for full range of motion without restriction. Opt for materials like cotton or moisture-wicking fabrics for optimal comfort.

A Supportive Surface: While mats are not essential for chair yoga, consider placing a **non-slip yoga mat** under your chair for added stability and cushioning, especially if practicing on hard floors.

Hydration Hero: Remember to stay hydrated! Keep a **reusable water bottle** handy to sip throughout your practice.

Optional Enhancements:

- **Yoga blocks:** These can provide support and assistance in various poses, especially if you have limited flexibility.
- **Straps:** Useful for extending your reach in certain stretches or improving alignment.
- **Meditation cushion:** If you wish to incorporate meditation into your practice, a cushion can elevate your hips and enhance comfort.
- **Relaxing music:** Set the mood with soothing music that promotes focus and mindfulness.

Setting the Stage:

- Choose a **well-lit, quiet space** free from distractions where you can move freely.

- Ensure **good ventilation** and a comfortable temperature.
- **Remove any obstacles** that might pose a tripping hazard.

Safety First:

- **Listen to your body** and avoid pushing yourself beyond your limits.
- **Take breaks** whenever needed.
- **Modify poses** to suit your individual needs and abilities.
- **Consult your doctor** before starting chair yoga if you have any concerns or pre-existing medical conditions.

With these simple essentials and a touch of enthusiasm, you're all set to embark on your transformative chair yoga journey! Remember, progress takes time and consistency. Embrace the gentle movements, enjoy the process, and discover the incredible benefits chair yoga has to offer.

Chapter 2

The Power of Having a developing mindset: Embracing Possibility in Chair Yoga

Imagine stepping into a chair yoga class filled with uncertainty. Your mind whispers: "You're too old for this," or "You'll never be as flexible as those others." These limiting beliefs, rooted in a fixed mindset, can hold you back from experiencing the incredible benefits of chair yoga. But what if you could unlock a different perspective, one that embraces challenges and views setbacks as opportunities for growth? This is the power of a developing mindset, and it has the potential to transform your chair yoga journey and, ultimately, your life.

Understanding the Mindset Landscape:

Our mindsets, whether fixed or growth, act as internal maps guiding our thoughts, actions, and ultimately, our results. In a **fixed mindset**, we believe our abilities are predetermined and immutable. Challenges become threats, mistakes solidify self-doubt, and progress feels impossible. Conversely, a **developing mindset** views abilities as malleable and nurtured through effort, learning, and experience. Challenges become opportunities to learn, mistakes become stepping stones, and progress becomes a celebrated journey.

developing mindset in Action: Your Chair Yoga Transformation

So, how does a developing mindset translate into your chair yoga practice? Imagine feeling stiffness in a pose. In a fixed mindset, you might give up, reinforcing the notion that flexibility is out of reach. But with a developing mindset, you view stiffness as a temporary hurdle. You explore modifications, seek guidance, and celebrate even small improvements in flexibility. This shift in perspective fuels motivation, fosters perseverance, and opens the door to continuous progress.

Beyond Flexibility: Unlocking the Full Potential of a developing mindset:

The benefits of a developing mindset extend far beyond physical improvements. Imagine experiencing self-doubt while attempting a new pose. In a fixed mindset, it might solidify negative self-talk. However, a developing mindset allows you to reframe self-doubt as a natural part of the learning process. You remind yourself that everyone starts somewhere and approach the pose with curiosity and a willingness to learn. This fosters self-compassion, enhances confidence, and fuels the joy of discovery within your practice.

Cultivating a developing mindset: Your Transformation Toolkit:

Embracing a developing mindset isn't about flipping a switch; it's a journey of self-discovery and mindful practice. Here are some tools to equip you on your path:

- **Challenge negative self-talk:** Recognize limiting beliefs and replace them with empowering affirmations.
- **Embrace challenges:** View them as opportunities to learn and grow, not insurmountable obstacles.
- **Celebrate small wins:** Acknowledge and celebrate every step forward, no matter how small.
- **Focus on effort:** Recognize that progress comes from dedicated practice, not just innate talent.
- **Learn from mistakes:** See them as valuable learning experiences, not failures.
- **Seek inspiration:** Surround yourself with individuals who embody a developing mindset.

Transformational Stories: Real-Life Inspiration

In this chapter, include inspiring stories of women over 60 who have transformed their lives through chair yoga and a developing mindset.

Share their challenges, their breakthroughs, and how they embraced the process. These stories serve as powerful testaments to the transformative power of shifting your perspective and celebrating the journey of growth.

The Relevance of a developing mindset in Chair Yoga for Women Over 60: Embracing Possibility and Overcoming Challenges

For women over 60, stepping into a chair yoga class can be an exciting prospect, but also potentially daunting. Ageist narratives that emphasize limitations and a fixed mindset can whisper, "You're too old," or "You'll never be flexible enough." But what if you could unlock a key that transforms your experience – the **developing mindset**? This chapter explores how embracing a developing mindset empowers women over 60 to navigate chair yoga with joy, conquer challenges, and achieve remarkable transformations.

Understanding the Mindset Landscape:

Our mindsets, whether fixed or growth, act as internal maps shaping our thoughts, actions, and ultimately, our results. In a **fixed mindset**, abilities are seen as static and unchangeable. Challenges become threats, mistakes solidify self-doubt, and progress feels impossible.

Conversely, a **developing mindset** views abilities as **malleable and nurtured through effort, learning, and experience**. Challenges become opportunities to learn, mistakes become stepping stones, and progress becomes a celebrated journey.

Why developing mindset Matters in Chair Yoga:

For women over 60, a developing mindset holds particular significance in chair yoga. It empowers you to:

- **Embrace Challenges, Not Fear Them:** Instead of viewing stiffness as a sign of inflexibility, you see it as a temporary hurdle to overcome with effort and modification. This fuels motivation and perseverance, transforming challenges into opportunities for growth.
- **Celebrate Small Wins:** A developing mindset shifts focus from the end goal to the joy of the journey. Even minor improvements in flexibility or strength

become stepping stones, fostering a sense of accomplishment and fueling continued practice.

- **Reframe Self-Doubt:** Negative self-talk, a common foe in a fixed mindset, loses its power. You recognize self-doubt as a natural part of the learning process and replace it with empowering affirmations, boosting confidence and self-compassion.
- **Find Joy in the Process:** With a developing mindset, the focus shifts from perfectionism to the inherent joy of movement and learning. You discover the fun in exploring new poses, experimenting with modifications, and celebrating your body's unique capabilities.

Cultivating a developing mindset: Your Toolkit:

Shifting to a developing mindset is a journey, not a destination. Here are some tools to equip you on your path:

- **Challenge Negative Self-Talk:** Identify limiting beliefs and replace them with affirmations like "I am capable of learning and growing."
- **Reframe Challenges:** Instead of "I can't do this," rephrase as "This is a challenge I can learn from."
- **Seek Inspiration:** Surround yourself with individuals who embody a developing mindset, like supportive classmates or inspiring instructors.
- **Focus on Effort:** Recognize that progress comes from dedicated practice, not just innate talent. Celebrate your effort, not just the outcome.
- **Learn from Mistakes:** View them as valuable learning experiences, not failures. Analyze what went wrong and apply the insights to future attempts.

Transformational Stories: Real-Life Inspiration:

In this chapter, include inspiring stories of women over 60 who have overcome challenges and achieved remarkable progress in chair yoga thanks to a developing mindset. Share how they confronted doubts, embraced learning, and celebrated their journeys. These real-life experiences serve as powerful testimonies to the transformative potential of mindset.

The Fixed Mindset vs. the developing mindset: Embracing Possibility in Chair Yoga

As you embark on your chair yoga journey, understanding the difference between a **fixed mindset** and a **developing mindset** can be crucial for overcoming challenges and celebrating progress. These contrasting mindsets shape how we perceive our abilities, approach challenges, and ultimately, determine our success.

The Fixed Mindset:

Imagine yourself entering a chair yoga class for the first time. A fixed mindset whispers anxieties: "You're too inflexible," "These poses are too difficult," or "It's too late to start something new." In a fixed mindset, your abilities are seen as **unchangeable and predetermined**. Challenges are viewed as threats, mistakes as setbacks, and progress feels limited. This can lead to:

- **Fear of new experiences:** Worried about failing, you might avoid trying challenging poses or attending classes.
- **Discouragement:** Mistakes become confirmation of your perceived limitations, leading to self-doubt and decreased motivation.
- **Focus on outcomes:** The pressure to achieve quick results overshadows the joy of learning and the journey of progress.

The developing mindset:

Now imagine approaching the same class with a developing mindset. You think: "This feels challenging, but I can learn and improve with practice." "Every mistake is an opportunity to learn and grow stronger." In a developing mindset, your abilities are seen as **malleable and nurtured through effort and experience**. Challenges are viewed as opportunities to learn, mistakes as stepping stones, and progress is celebrated every step of the way. This can lead to:

- **Embrace of challenges:** You view them as opportunities to learn and grow, fostering curiosity and a willingness to experiment.
- **Resilience:** Mistakes become learning experiences, motivating you to try again with a different approach.
- **Focus on the process:** The joy of movement, exploration, and personal growth become central to your experience.

Chair Yoga and the developing mindset:

For women over 60, a developing mindset can be particularly transformative in chair yoga. It empowers you to:

- **Embrace stiffness:** Instead of seeing it as a fixed limitation, you view it as a temporary hurdle to overcome with effort and modifications.
- **Celebrate small wins:** Even minor improvements in flexibility or strength become stepping stones, fostering a sense

of accomplishment and fueling continued practice.

- **Reframe self-doubt:** Negative self-talk loses its power. You recognize it as a natural part of the learning process and replace it with empowering affirmations.
- **Find joy in the process:** The focus shifts from perfectionism to the inherent joy of movement and learning. You discover the fun in exploring new poses, experimenting with modifications, and celebrating your body's unique capabilities.

Cultivating a developing mindset:

Shifting to a developing mindset is a journey, not a destination. Here are some practices to help you on your way:

- **Challenge negative self-talk:** Identify limiting beliefs and replace them with affirmations like "I am capable of learning and growing."

- **Reframe challenges:** Instead of "I can't do this," rephrase as "This is a challenge I can learn from."
- **Seek inspiration:** Surround yourself with individuals who embody a developing mindset, like supportive classmates or inspiring instructors.
- **Focus on effort:** Recognize that progress comes from dedicated practice, not just innate talent. Celebrate your effort, not just the outcome.
- **Learn from mistakes:** View them as valuable learning experiences, not failures. Analyze what went wrong and apply the insights to future attempts.

Remember, you are not limited by your age or perceived limitations. By embracing a developing mindset, you open the door to endless possibilities in chair yoga and beyond. Celebrate the journey of progress, one gentle pose at a time.

Fixed vs. developing mindset in Chair Yoga

Imagine yourself stepping into a chair yoga class. How your mind interprets the experience depends on your dominant mindset: fixed or growth. Let's see how these contrasting mindsets manifest in relatable scenarios for women over 60:

Fixed Mindset:

- **Doris:** Her heart races with anxiety. "Everyone else looks so flexible," she thinks, "I'll never be able to do those poses." Doris avoids challenging poses, convinced she's "too old" or "not good enough." Discouragement sets in, and she contemplates quitting.
- **Margaret:** During Warrior Pose, she feels tightness in her hamstrings. "See, I'm too inflexible," she scoffs, instantly deflating. Margaret focuses on the discomfort, feeling discouraged and questioning her ability to continue.

- **Eleanor:** Struggling with a balance pose, she stumbles slightly. "I knew I shouldn't have tried," she thinks, feeling embarrassed and defeated. Eleanor labels the mistake as proof of her limitations, diminishing her confidence and motivation.

developing mindset:

- **Brenda:** Feeling a flutter of nervousness, Brenda tells herself, "This is new, and that's okay. I'll try my best." She observes others with curiosity, noticing modifications they use. Brenda embraces the challenge, finding joy in the act of trying.
- **Helen:** Tightness in her hamstrings doesn't surprise her. "This is a chance to work on my flexibility," she thinks, adjusting her stance for a deeper stretch. Helen focuses on the breath and sensation, viewing the challenge as an opportunity to learn and grow.

- **Susan:** Losing her balance momentarily, Susan chuckles and regains her footing. "Oops, that was wobbly!" she thinks, "But I caught myself." Susan laughs it off, seeing the stumble as a learning experience, not a failure.

The Impact of Mindset:

These examples illustrate how mindsets shape our experiences. A fixed mindset breeds negativity, fear, and self-doubt, hindering progress and enjoyment. Conversely, a developing mindset fosters curiosity, resilience, and self-compassion, creating a foundation for learning, growth, and lasting joy in chair yoga.

Remember:

- You are not defined by your current limitations. A developing mindset allows you to see them as temporary hurdles, not insurmountable obstacles.
- Every stumble, every ache, is an opportunity to learn and refine your

practice. Embrace the journey, not just the
destination.
- Celebrate small wins, no matter how
  seemingly insignificant. They are stepping
  stones on your path to progress and
  self-discovery.

By adopting a developing mindset, you unlock the true potential of chair yoga, transforming it from a mere exercise routine into a journey of self-empowerment and joyful discovery. So, step onto your mat with curiosity and a willingness to learn, and watch your possibilities unfold, one gentle pose at a time.

Blossoming Through Chair Yoga: The developing mindset Advantage

Imagine yourself embarking on a chair yoga journey. As you step onto the mat, your mind whispers questions. Will you embrace the possibilities, or let limiting beliefs hold you back? Enter the **developing mindset**, a powerful tool that unlocks the transformative potential of chair yoga for women over 60. Let's explore the bountiful benefits it offers:

1. Enhanced Motivation and Perseverance:

- Fixed mindset: "I'm too stiff, I won't improve."
- developing mindset: "This pose feels challenging, but I can work on it with practice."

A fixed mindset sets limitations, while a developing mindset sees challenges as opportunities. You're driven by the **joy of learning** and the belief that progress takes time and effort. Minor improvements become stepping stones, fueling your desire to continue your practice.

2. Increased Confidence and Self-Compassion:

- Fixed mindset: "Everyone else is more flexible, I'm not good enough."
- developing mindset: "Everyone starts somewhere, I'm proud of my effort."

The fixed mindset breeds self-doubt, while the developing mindset fosters **self-compassion**. You learn to recognize and reframe negative thoughts, replacing them with **empowering affirmations**. Instead of judging yourself, you celebrate your unique abilities and progress.

3. Greater Enjoyment and Flexibility:

- Fixed mindset: "This pose is painful, I should stick to the easy ones."
- developing mindset: "I can experiment with modifications to make this pose more comfortable and effective."

With a fixed mindset, discomfort discourages exploration. With a developing mindset, you **embrace experimentation**, trying different modifications and props to find what works for you. This open-minded approach enhances your practice, making it both enjoyable and effective.

4. Improved Well-being and Sense of Accomplishment:

- Fixed mindset: "I'll never be as flexible as others, what's the point?"
- developing mindset: "Every breath, every pose is a step towards feeling stronger and more balanced."

The fixed mindset focuses on achieving a distant goal, neglecting the journey. The developing mindset celebrates **gradual progress**, noticing improvements in strength, flexibility, and balance. This ongoing sense of accomplishment contributes to your overall well-being and motivates you to continue.

5. Embracing Change and Lifelong Learning:

- Fixed mindset: "I'm too old to learn new things."
- developing mindset: "This practice keeps me learning and growing, regardless of age."

A fixed mindset fears change and new experiences. The developing mindset sees them as opportunities for growth. You learn to **embrace challenges**, knowing that learning never stops. This empowers you to adapt to new poses, routines, and even life's unexpected turns with resilience and flexibility.

Remember:

The developing mindset is not a magic switch, but a journey of self-discovery. Here are some tips to cultivate it:

- **Challenge negative self-talk:** Identify limiting beliefs and replace them with positive affirmations.

- **Celebrate small wins:** Acknowledge and celebrate every step forward, no matter how small.
- **Focus on effort:** Recognize that progress comes from dedicated practice, not just innate talent.
- **Learn from mistakes:** See them as valuable learning experiences, not failures.
- **Seek inspiration:** Surround yourself with individuals who embody a developing mindset.

By embracing a developing mindset, you unlock the true potential of chair yoga, transforming it from a mere exercise routine into a journey of self-empowerment, lifelong learning, and joyful discovery. So, step onto your mat with an open mind and a willingness to learn, and watch your possibilities unfold, one gentle pose at a time.

Chapter 3

Gentle Warm-Up Exercises for Chair Yoga

Preparing Body and Mind

Before diving into your chair yoga practice, a mindful warm-up is crucial to prepare your body and mind for movement. These gentle exercises help activate muscles, increase blood flow, and focus your attention, leading to a more enjoyable and beneficial experience.

Preparation:

- Find a quiet space with adequate ventilation and comfortable lighting.
- Wear loose, breathable clothing that allows easy movement.
- Remove any jewelry or accessories that might hinder your practice.

- Sit comfortably in your chair with your
  feet flat on the floor and back straight.

Warm-Up Exercises:

1. Neck Rolls:

- Gently roll your head in a circular motion,
  first clockwise and then
  counter-clockwise, 5 times each direction.
- Feel the tension releasing in your neck
  and shoulders.

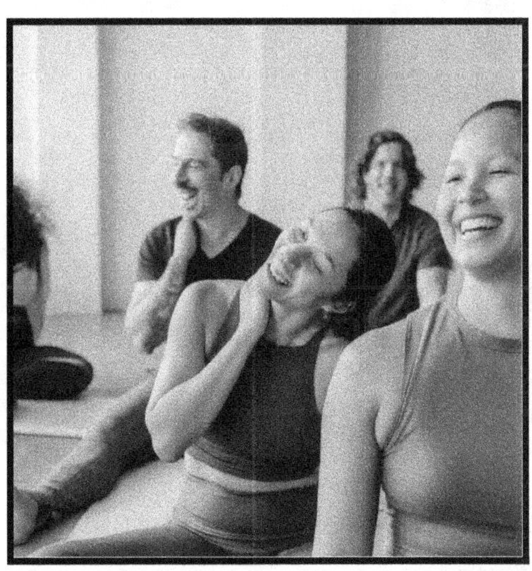

2. Shoulder Shrugs:

- Slowly lift your shoulders towards your ears, hold for a moment, and then release them down with a relaxed sigh. Repeat 5 times

3. Arm Circles:

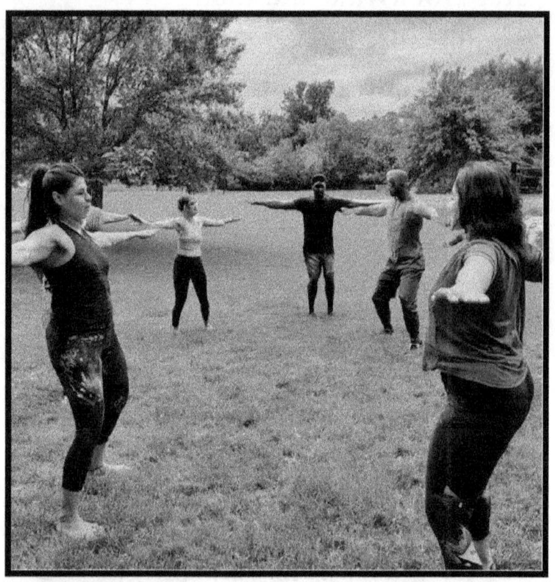

- Extend your arms straight out to the sides, palms facing up. Make small circles

forward and then backward, 5 times each
direction.

4. Wrist Circles:

- With your hands relaxed and fingers
  together, make small circles forward and
  then backward, 5 times each direction.

5. Gentle Twists:

- Place your right hand on your right knee and gently twist your upper body to the left. Hold for a few breaths, then repeat on the other side.

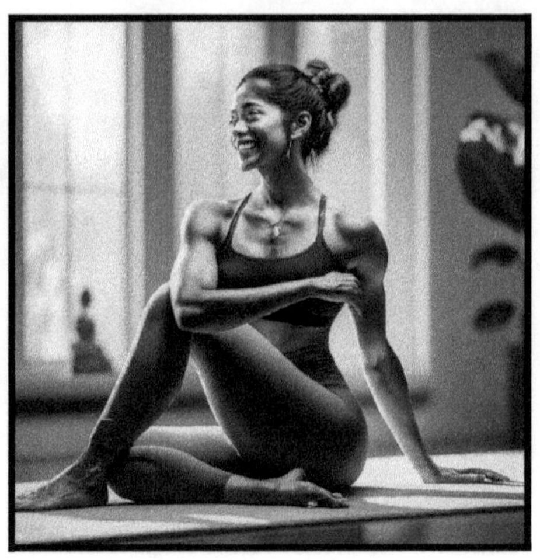

6. Ankle Circles:

- Rotate your ankles in clockwise and counter-clockwise circles, 5 times each direction. Feel the movement travel up your calves.

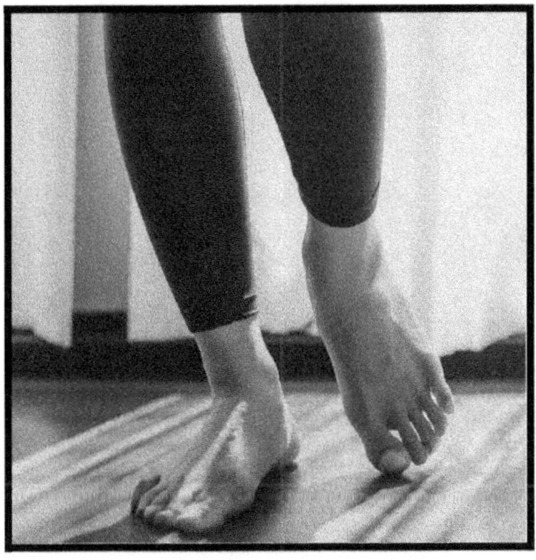

7. Deep Breaths:

- Close your eyes and take 5 deep, slow breaths in through your nose and out through your mouth. Focus on the rise and fall of your chest and abdomen.

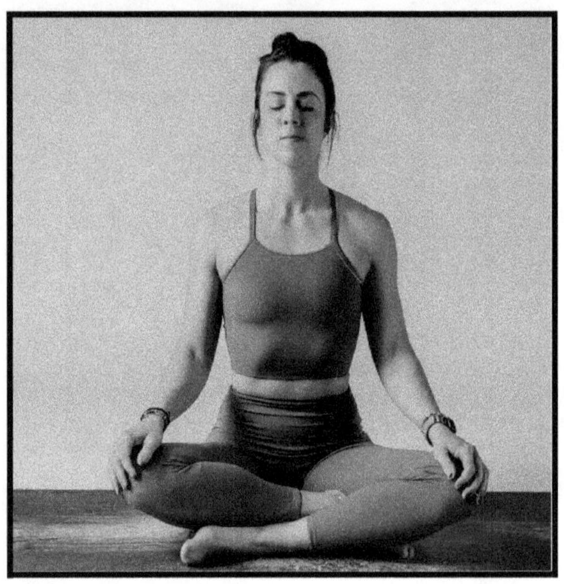

Additional Tips:

- Listen to your body and modify any exercises as needed.
- Don't force movements that cause pain or discomfort.

- Focus on slow, controlled movements and synchronize your breath with each exercise.
- Smile and enjoy the process of preparing your body and mind for your practice.

Remember:

Taking a few minutes for a gentle warm-up sets the stage for a safe, enjoyable, and effective chair yoga experience. Let these exercises help you connect with your body, quiet your mind, and be fully present for your practice.

Protecting your body is essential in any physical activity, including chair yoga. Here are some key points to remember:

Before you start:

- **Consult your doctor:** Especially if you have any pre-existing medical conditions, injuries, or limitations.
- **Choose the right chair:** Opt for a sturdy, armless chair with a flat seat and a back that allows you to sit comfortably with your feet flat on the floor.
- **Wear appropriate clothing:** Loose, breathable clothing allows for easy movement and prevents chafing.
- **Listen to your body:** Don't push yourself beyond your limits and modify poses as needed. Pain is a signal to stop or adjust.

During your practice:

- **Maintain proper form:** Pay attention to alignment, joint positioning, and core engagement to avoid injury.

- **Focus on mindful movement:** Be present in each pose and avoid rushing or forcing your body into uncomfortable positions.
- **Use breathwork:** Synchronize your breath with your movements to enhance focus and regulate your heart rate.
- **Stay hydrated:** Drink plenty of water before, during, and after your practice to avoid dehydration.
- **Take breaks:** Don't be afraid to rest and recover when needed.

Additional tips:

- **Warm-up and cool down:** Prepare your body with gentle warm-up exercises and cool down with stretches to prevent muscle soreness.
- **Use props:** Blocks, straps, and cushions can help modify poses and provide support for specific needs.
- **Be patient:** Progress takes time, so don't get discouraged if you don't see results immediately. Celebrate small improvements and focus on your journey.

- **Choose an instructor you trust:** If you're new to chair yoga, consider attending a class led by a qualified and experienced instructor who can provide guidance and personalized feedback.

Remember: Protecting your body is key to enjoying the benefits of chair yoga for years to come. By following these guidelines and listening to your body, you can create a safe and rewarding practice that enhances your physical and mental well-being.

Paying Attention to Health Problems in Chair Yoga: A Proactive Approach

While chair yoga offers numerous benefits for women over 60, it's crucial to remain aware of potential health concerns and how to navigate them safely. Here are some key points to remember:

Before you start:

- **Listen to your body:** Pay attention to any pain, discomfort, or dizziness you experience during daily activities. These could be signs of underlying health issues that require medical attention before starting chair yoga.
- **Communicate with your doctor:** Discuss your intention to practice chair yoga and any relevant medical conditions you might have. Your doctor can advise on modifications or precautions necessary for your specific situation.
- **Know your limitations:** Be honest about your current physical abilities and

exercise history. Start slowly and gradually increase the intensity and duration of your practice as you gain strength and flexibility.

During your practice:

- **Be mindful of pain:** Pain is a signal from your body that something is wrong. If you experience sharp pain, stop the pose immediately and rest. Do not push through pain, as it can lead to injury.
- **Pay attention to dizziness:** If you feel dizzy or lightheaded, stop the pose, sit down, and rest. Take deep breaths and wait until the feeling passes before continuing.
- **Monitor your heart rate:** If you have heart conditions, monitor your heart rate during your practice. If it becomes too high, take a break or stop the practice altogether.
- **Communicate with your instructor:** If you participate in a chair yoga class, inform the instructor about any health

concerns you have and don't hesitate to ask for modifications or clarifications on poses.

Additional tips:

- **Start with gentle poses:** Don't begin with advanced or strenuous poses, especially if you're new to chair yoga. Focus on basic movements that build strength and flexibility gradually.
- **Use props wisely:** Blocks, straps, and cushions can help you maintain proper form, modify poses, and prevent strain. Don't hesitate to utilize them for added support and comfort.
- **Hydrate adequately:** Drink plenty of water before, during, and after your practice to stay hydrated and prevent dehydration, which can worsen certain health conditions.
- **Listen to your body and take breaks:** Don't be afraid to rest when you need to. Pushing yourself too hard can lead to

fatigue, injury, or worsen existing health problems.

Remember:

Paying attention to your body and health is crucial for a safe and enjoyable chair yoga experience. By communicating with your doctor, respecting your limitations, and modifying poses as needed, you can maximize the benefits of chair yoga while minimizing risks.

Chapter 4

16 Simple Chair Yoga Poses for Your Daily Routine

Integrating yoga into your daily routine takes dedication and mindful planning, but the rewards are immense. Here's how you can turn your intentions into consistent practice:

Start Small and Be Realistic:

- Don't overwhelm yourself by aiming for hour-long sessions daily. Begin with 5-10 minute practices and gradually increase duration as you build stamina and enthusiasm.
- Choose a specific time that works for you, be it early morning, lunchtime, or before bed. Consistency is key, so pick a time you're most likely to stick to.

Find Your Yoga Style:

- Explore different styles like Hatha, Vinyasa, or Chair Yoga to discover what resonates with your body and preferences. Consider online resources, free classes, or studio trials.
- Remember, there's no "one size fits all" approach. Choose a style that feels enjoyable and physically attainable.

Create a Dedicated Space:

- Even a small corner with a yoga mat or comfortable rug can become your sanctuary. Ensure good lighting, ventilation, and minimal distractions.
- Having a designated space reinforces the association between the space and your yoga practice, making it easier to transition into mindfulness.

Prepare Your Mind and Body:

- Set the mood with soft music, aromatherapy, or inspirational quotes.

Take a few minutes to quiet your mind through meditation or deep breathing exercises.

- Gentle stretches or warm-up activities help prepare your body for movement and prevent injuries.

Embrace Modifications:

- Don't compare yourself to others! Every body is unique, and poses can be adapted to your limitations. Use blocks, straps, or chairs for support as needed.
- Listen to your body and prioritize safety over pushing yourself into discomfort. Remember, progress takes time and mindful practice.

Make it Fun and Social:

- Practice with a friend or join a virtual yoga community to create accountability and share the experience.
- If you enjoy music, choose playlists that energize or relax you during your practice.

- Reward yourself for achieving milestones, like completing a longer session or mastering a new pose.

Track Your Progress:

- Journal about your practice, noting your mood, physical sensations, and progress. This helps stay motivated and identify areas to focus on.
- Track your sessions using apps or calendars to maintain consistency and celebrate your growing commitment.

Most importantly, remember:

- Yoga is a journey, not a destination. Be patient with yourself, enjoy the process, and focus on the present moment.
- Consistency is key to reaping the benefits of yoga. Even short, regular practices can significantly improve your well-being.

By following these tips and tailoring them to your specific needs and preferences, you can successfully integrate yoga into your daily routine and unlock its transformative power.

16 gentle chair yoga poses you can easily incorporate into your daily routine:

Warm-Up (5-10 minutes):

1. **Neck Rolls:** Gently roll your head in a circle, first clockwise and then counter-clockwise, 5 times each direction.
2. **Shoulder Shrugs:** Lift your shoulders towards your ears, hold for a moment, and then release them down with a relaxed sigh. Repeat 5 times.
3. **Arm Circles:** Extend your arms straight out to the sides, palms facing up. Make small circles forward and then backward, 5 times each direction.
4. **Wrist Circles:** With your hands relaxed and fingers together, make small circles forward and then backward, 5 times each direction.
5. **Gentle Twists:** Place your right hand on your right knee and gently twist your upper body to the left. Hold for a few breaths, then repeat on the other side.

Standing Poses (5 minutes):

6. **Raised Arms:** Stand behind your chair, hold the backrest for balance, and lift your arms overhead. Breathe deeply and feel your torso lengthen. Hold for 5 breaths.

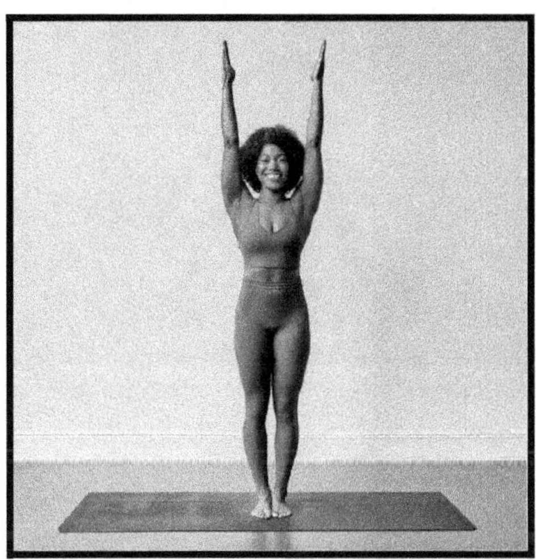

7. **Heel Raises:** Stand behind your chair with your hands on the backrest. Rise up onto your toes, hold for a few seconds, and lower back down. Repeat 10 times.
8. **Side Bends:** Stand behind your chair, hold the backrest with one hand, and reach the other arm overhead. Gently bend to the

side, stretching your waist and obliques.
Hold for 5 breaths each side.

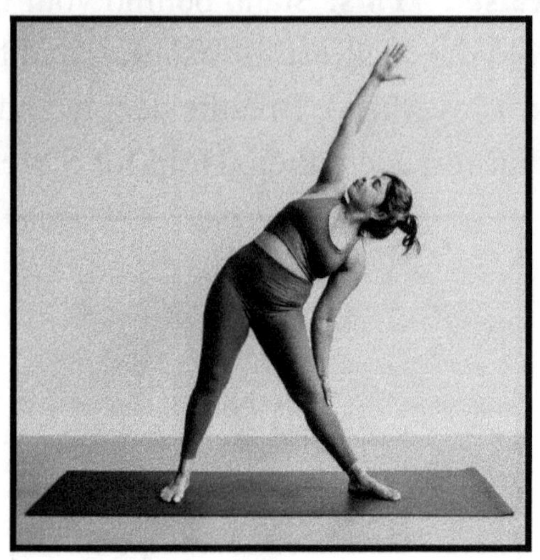

Seated Poses (10 minutes):

9. **Seated Spinal Twists:** Sit tall in your chair, hands on your knees. Twist your upper body to one side, hold for a few breaths, and then repeat on the other side.

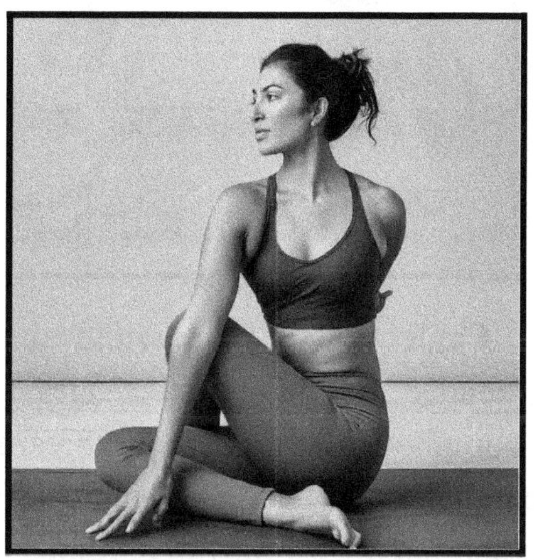

10. **Cat-Cow Poses:** Sit tall with hands on knees. On an inhale, arch your back like a cat, looking up. On an exhale, round your back like a cow, tucking your chin to your chest. Repeat 5 times.

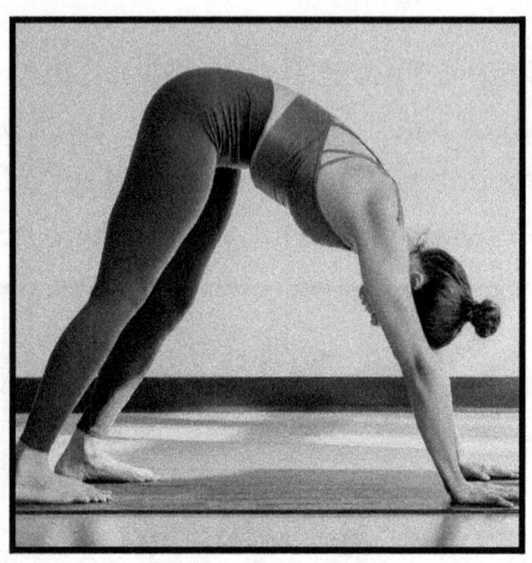

11. **Eagle Arms:** Sit tall with your arms extended straight out to the sides. Bend your elbows and bring your forearms parallel to the floor, one on top of the other. Interlace your fingers and gaze at your fingertips. Hold for 5 breaths and repeat on the other side.

12. **Leg Extensions:** Sit tall and extend one leg straight out in front of you. Hold for a few breaths and then switch legs. Repeat 5 times each side.

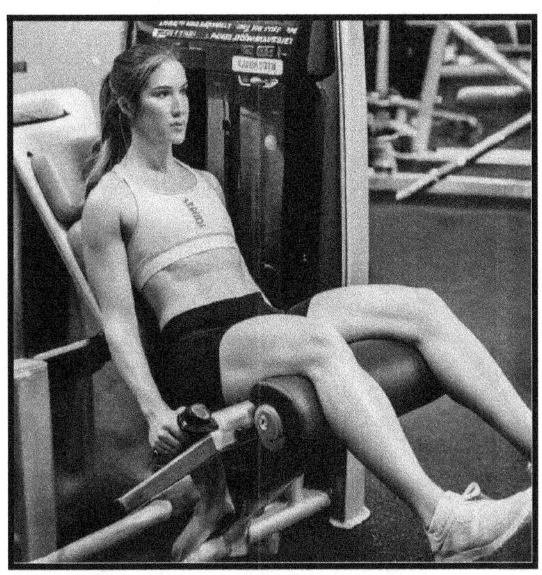

Cool-Down (5 minutes):

13.   **Seated Forward Bends:** Sit tall and gently fold forward, reaching towards your toes or the floor. Breathe deeply and hold for 5 breaths.
14.   **Ankle Circles:** Rotate your ankles in clockwise and counter-clockwise circles, 5 times each direction.

15. **Deep Breaths:** Close your eyes and take 5 deep, slow breaths in through your nose and out through your mouth. Focus on the rise and fall of your chest and abdomen.

16. **Relaxation:** Sit quietly in your chair and allow your body to relax. Focus on your breath and appreciate the benefits of your practice.

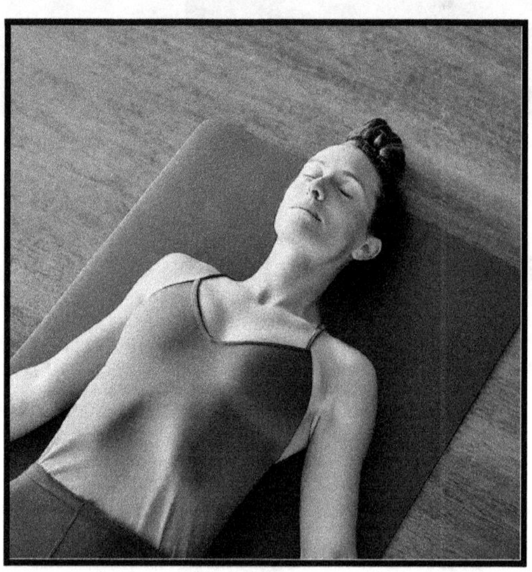

Remember:

- Modify poses as needed to suit your physical limitations.
- Listen to your body and take breaks as needed.
- Focus on your breath and enjoy the movement.
- Start slowly and gradually increase the duration and intensity of your practice as you become stronger and more flexible.

Chapter 5

12 Seated Cardio Workouts for Weight Loss (and Overall Fitness) for Women Over 60:

While chair yoga itself isn't specifically designed for weight loss, incorporating these seated cardio workouts into your routine can help boost your calorie burn and support weight management alongside a healthy diet. Remember, the key is to find activities you enjoy and can do consistently. Here are 12 options:

Low-Impact Workouts:

1. **Seated Arm Circles:** Forward and backward circles with both arms simultaneously, then alternate arms. Gradually increase speed for higher intensity.

2. **Heel Taps:** Tap heels alternately on the floor, gradually increasing speed and height of taps.
3. **Leg Extensions:** Straighten one leg out then bring it back, alternating legs. Add ankle weights for more resistance.
4. **Seated Marches:** March legs in the air, alternating knees, gradually increasing speed.
5. **Chair Squats:** Stand up from a seated position, hold for a moment, then sit back down slowly. Start with minimal squats and gradually increase depth.

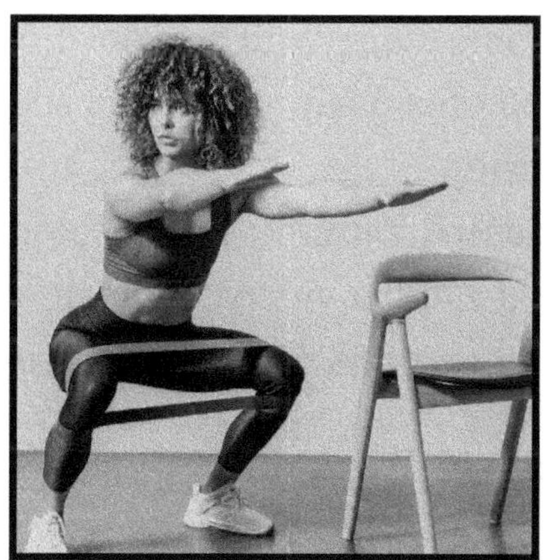

6. **Seated Swimming:** Pretend you're swimming, moving your arms in freestyle or butterfly motions.

Moderate-Impact Workouts:

7. **Jumping Jacks (Seated Version):** Raise your hands overhead and tap your knees with your hands while seated, increasing speed and intensity.
8. **Seated Boxercise:** Punch the air with alternating arms, add wrist weights for more challenge.
9. **Stair Climber (Chair Exercise):** Mimic climbing stairs with leg movements while seated on a chair, increasing speed and intensity.
10. **Seated Zumba:** Follow along with seated Zumba videos or create your own seated versions of Zumba moves.

Higher-Impact Workouts:

11. **Burpees (Seated Variation):** Stand up from a seated position, clap your hands

overhead, then quickly sit back down. Do as many as you can within your comfort zone.

12.   **Jumping Jacks (Modified):** Raise your hands overhead while seated, then lift your bottom off the chair momentarily for a mini-jump. Gradually increase height and speed.

Additional Tips:

- Warm up before your workout with gentle stretches and light movement.
- Cool down afterwards with static stretches and deep breathing.
- Modify exercises as needed to suit your fitness level and limitations.
- Listen to your body and take breaks when needed.
- Consult your doctor before starting any new exercise program.
- Combine these seated exercises with standing exercises or other forms of activity for a well-rounded workout plan.

Remember, consistency is key. By incorporating these seated cardio workouts into your routine, along with healthy eating habits, you can improve your overall fitness and contribute to weight management efforts in a safe and enjoyable way.

Chapter 6

15-minute chair yoga

Warm-Up (5 minutes):

- **Neck Rolls:** Gently roll your head in a circle, first clockwise and then counter-clockwise, 5 times each direction.
- **Shoulder Shrugs:** Lift your shoulders towards your ears, hold for a moment, and then release them down with a relaxed sigh. Repeat 5 times.
- **Arm Circles:** Extend your arms straight out to the sides, palms facing up. Make small circles forward and then backward, 5 times each direction.
- **Wrist Circles:** With your hands relaxed and fingers together, make small circles

forward and then backward, 5 times each direction.

- **Ankle Circles:** Rotate your ankles in clockwise and counter-clockwise circles, 5 times each direction.

Seated Poses (7 minutes):

- **Seated Cat-Cow Poses:** Sit tall with hands on knees. On an inhale, arch your back like a cat, looking up. On an exhale, round your back like a cow, tucking your chin to your chest. Repeat 5 times.
- **Eagle Arms:** Sit tall with your arms extended straight out to the sides. Bend your elbows and bring your forearms parallel to the floor, one on top of the other. Interlace your fingers and gaze at your fingertips. Hold for 5 breaths and repeat on the other side.
- **Seated Spinal Twists:** Place your right hand on your right knee and gently twist your upper body to the left. Hold for a few breaths, then repeat on the other side. (2 sets)

- **Leg Extensions:** Sit tall and extend one leg straight out in front of you. Hold for a few breaths and then switch legs. Repeat 5 times each side.

Cool-Down (3 minutes):

- **Seated Forward Bends:** Sit tall and gently fold forward, reaching towards your toes or the floor. Breathe deeply and hold for 5 breaths.
- **Deep Breaths:** Close your eyes and take 5 deep, slow breaths in through your nose and out through your mouth. Focus on the rise and fall of your chest and abdomen.

Modifications:

- Use a chair with a back for support if needed.
- Sit on a cushion or rolled-up towel for added comfort.
- Use blocks or straps to assist you in reaching deeper into poses.

- Listen to your body and modify poses as needed.

Tips:

- Focus on your breath and connect with your body throughout the sequence.
- Move slowly and mindfully, feeling each stretch and movement.
- Don't push yourself beyond your limits.
- You can repeat this sequence several times a week for a quick and effective yoga practice.

Enjoy your chair yoga journey!

Chapter 7

Holistic wellness diet

A holistic wellness diet focuses on nourishing your body with whole, unprocessed foods to promote both physical and mental well-being. It goes beyond mere calorie counting and dietary trends, emphasizing mindful eating and an intuitive relationship with food. Here are some key principles of a holistic wellness diet for women over 60:

Prioritize Whole Foods:

- **Fruits and vegetables:** Choose diverse colors and varieties for an abundance of vitamins, minerals, and antioxidants. Focus on seasonal and locally grown options whenever possible.

- **Whole grains:** Opt for brown rice, quinoa, oats, and whole-wheat bread instead of refined grains for more fiber and nutrients.
- **Lean protein:** Include sources like fish, poultry, beans, lentils, and nuts for essential amino acids.
- **Healthy fats:** Incorporate avocado, olive oil, and fatty fish for satiety, heart health, and brain function.

Minimize Processed Foods:

- **Limit sugary drinks:** Opt for water, herbal teas, or diluted fruit juices instead of soda, sugary coffees, and artificial sweeteners.
- **Reduce refined carbohydrates:** Avoid white bread, pastries, and processed snacks that cause blood sugar spikes and crashes.
- **Beware of unhealthy fats:** Limit saturated and trans fats found in fried foods, processed meats, and commercially baked goods.

Listen to Your Body:

- **Practice mindful eating:** Pay attention to hunger and satiety cues, eating slowly and savoring your food.
- **Hydrate adequately:** Drink plenty of water throughout the day to stay energized and support digestion.
- **Consider food sensitivities:** Pay attention to how certain foods make you feel and adjust your diet accordingly.
- **Embrace variety:** Explore different flavors and textures to keep your meals interesting and enjoyable.

Additional Tips:

- **Cook at home more often:** This gives you control over ingredients and portion sizes.
- **Incorporate fermented foods:** Yogurt, kimchi, and sauerkraut provide beneficial probiotics for gut health.

- **Season meals with herbs and spices:**
  These add flavor without relying on
  excessive salt.
- **Find support:** Join a cooking class, seek
  nutrition counseling, or connect with
  like-minded individuals for motivation.

Remember:

- A holistic wellness diet is not a restrictive
  regimen but a mindful approach to
  nourishing your body with respect and
  understanding.
- It's a journey, not a destination, so be
  patient, experiment, and celebrate your
  progress.
- This information is intended for general
  knowledge and should not be considered a
  substitute for professional medical advice.
  Consult a healthcare professional for
  personalized dietary guidance.

By embracing these principles, you can cultivate
a holistic wellness diet that supports your unique

needs and empowers you to thrive in body and mind.

Conclusion

Embracing a Joyful Journey with Chair Yoga

As you reach the culmination of this exploration of chair yoga, remember that you've embarked on a journey, not just completed a book. The poses etched within these pages are but stepping stones on a path towards strength, flexibility, peace, and most importantly, **joy**.

This journey will unfold differently for each of you. Your unique story, your body's whispers, and your spirit's desires will guide your practice. Embrace the modifications, celebrate the small victories, and find laughter in the moments of wobbly balance.

Remember, chair yoga is more than just physical movement. It's a doorway to **self-discovery**. As you connect with your breath, lengthen your spine, and find stability in each pose, you'll also discover resilience, self-compassion, and a renewed sense of possibility.

Let this practice be a source of **joy**. Embrace the moments of quiet focus, the laughter shared with friends in class, and the newfound confidence that radiates from within. As you step off your mat, carry that joy with you into every aspect of your life.

Here are some concluding thoughts to leave your readers with:

- Share your chair yoga journey! Inspire others by sharing your story, experiences, and newfound joys.
- Continue exploring! There's always more to learn and discover in the world of yoga.
- Nurture your well-being! Beyond chair yoga, explore healthy habits that nourish your body and mind.
- Most importantly, **never stop embracing joy!** Find it in movement, in stillness, and in every precious moment of your life.

May chair yoga be a constant companion on your journey towards a life filled with strength, flexibility, peace, and most importantly, **joy**.

Namaste.

Key Takeaways

Benefits:

- **Strength and Flexibility:** Chair yoga helps maintain and improve muscle strength and joint flexibility, promoting better balance and mobility.
- **Peace and Joy:** The practice incorporates mindfulness and breathwork, fostering relaxation and stress reduction, leading to greater peace and overall well-being.
- **Empowerment and Self-Discovery:** Adapting poses to suit your needs and limitations builds confidence and self-care, leading to a deeper understanding of your body and its potential.
- **Community and Connection:** Sharing the practice with others encourages social connection and support, adding a fun and uplifting dimension to your journey.

Key Principles:

- **Listen to your body:** Modify poses as needed and prioritize pain-free movement.
- **Focus on form and proper alignment:** Ensure safe and effective practice for maximum benefits.
- **Embrace mindful movement:** Connect with your breath and be present in each pose.
- **Make it enjoyable:** Explore different styles and find practices that spark joy and motivation.
- **Consistency is key:** Regular practice, even for short periods, yields greater results over time.

Actionable Advice:

- Consult your doctor before starting any new exercise program.
- Consider working with a qualified chair yoga instructor, especially if you are new to yoga or have specific health concerns.
- Start slowly and gradually increase the duration and intensity of your practice.

- Explore online resources, join virtual classes, or attend local workshops to expand your knowledge and practice.
- Find a comfortable and dedicated space for your practice.
- Share your journey with friends and family to encourage each other and stay accountable.
- Most importantly, celebrate your progress, embrace the joy of movement, and enjoy the transformation chair yoga brings to your life!

Remember: Chair yoga is an accessible and transformative practice for women over 60, offering a pathway to strength, flexibility, peace, and joyful living. Embrace the journey, personalize your practice, and discover the power within you!

Bonus

https://screenpal.com/watch/cZnIDbVdkfM

Video link for tutorials

Dear Helen Talbott

I'm thrilled to share my new book, **Chair Yoga for Women Over 60: Discover Strength, Flexibility, Peace, and Embrace Joy**, which I believe could greatly benefit you or someone you know.

This book is specifically designed for women over 60 who are looking for a gentle and effective way to improve their fitness, flexibility, and wellbeing. Whether you're a complete beginner or have some yoga experience, **Chair Yoga for Women Over 60** offers a safe and accessible practice that can be done entirely from a chair.

In the book, you'll find:

- **Easy-to-follow poses:** Illustrated instructions and modifications ensure you can practice safely and effectively at your own pace.

- **Focus on strength and flexibility:** Build balance, coordination, and core strength while increasing your range of motion.
- **Mindfulness and stress reduction:** Discover techniques to relax, de-stress, and cultivate inner peace.
- **Joyful movement:** Experience the physical and emotional benefits of gentle yoga in a supportive and encouraging environment.

I'm confident that **Chair Yoga for Women Over 60** can be a valuable resource for you or someone you know. To gain valuable insights from your perspective, I'd be honored if you would consider providing a review on . Your honest feedback would be incredibly helpful in spreading the word about this accessible and empowering practice.

- What aspects of the book did you find most helpful or informative?
- Did the poses and instructions feel clear and easy to follow?

- Did you find the focus on strength, flexibility, and mindfulness beneficial?
- Would you recommend this book to other women over 60?

Thank you for considering my request. I truly appreciate your time and feedback.

Warmly,

Helen Talbott